Getting Rid of Cellulite
in
10-Days

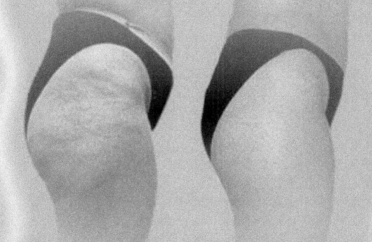

One Simple Step Does It!

Dr. Leland Benton

TABLE OF CONTENTS

Getting Rid of Cellulite in 10-Days
One Simple Step Does it!
©Copyright 2012 Dr. Leland Benton

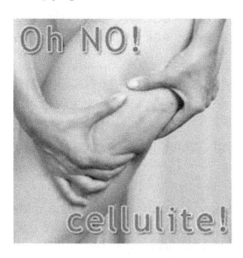

Introduction – Knowledge is Power Only When It Is Applied!

I read an article the other day titled..."Economy Squeezes the American Dream". It talked about the current economy's effect on the "American Dream."

From the very first sentence, I knew that the writer knew NOTHING about what the American dream was.

The very first sentence of the article was..."Work hard, play by the rules and tomorrow will be better than today." AMAZING!

Are you kidding me, I thought? The "work hard" part I got. It's a necessity to be able to live your dream lifestyle no matter where you live.

But, "play by the rules and tomorrow will be better than today." Excuse me, but that is pure unadulterated garbage! Here is what happens when you play by the rules....

> 1. You go to college and spend a ridiculous amount of money on a degree you in most cases will never use or

4

need. *I know; I have ten years of college and five degrees and left UCLA in 1980 with almost a quarter of a million dollars in student loan debt.*

2. You get a job that pays you little, but forces you to work 50 to 70 hours per week to make ends meet. *Sound familiar?*

3. You most likely have no job security and a boss and employer that cares little about you. *"You aren't family; get over it" is what they told me.*

4. You get the "privilege" of taking one vacation a year if you are lucky. *But you have very little disposable income to take a vacation!*

5. You work until you are at least 65 and possibly longer so that you can have just enough money to live out the rest of your days. Plus you no longer get a gold watch and you are lucky to get a pat on your head and a thank you. *Yeah, some American dream, right?*

Sound like the "American Dream" to you? Sounds more like a nightmare to me.

If you "play by the rules," that is a pretty likely scenario for you! Truth is, the article may have had good intentions, but was WAY off.

Those that have been able to live the "American Dream," or to live their dream lifestyle no matter where they are from, have never played by the rules.

Yes, hard work has always been a required element to living out your dream lifestyle. But those that have dream lifestyles almost always create their own rules.

They are what's called "self-made."

In fact, of the 15 wealthiest people in the world as of 2008, 10 of them are self made and 5 of them inherited the money.

Of the 10 that are self made billionaires, a whopping 9 are high school or college dropouts!

Am I preaching against getting an education? No; but if you want to live your dream lifestyle, you have to take charge of your own life.

You have to make your own rules. And, you have to make things happen for yourself.

Many years ago, after being let go from my job 3 weeks before Christmas with a baby on the way and by an employer who cared little about me or my family no matter how hard I worked, I took charge of my life.

Today... I work when I want to. I play when I want to. I vacation when I want to. I can afford the things that I want. I am my own boss!

And....I definitely DO NOT play by the rules. I make my own.

If you want to play by the rules, go ahead. But, don't expect any sort of dream lifestyle out of it.

If you want to start taking control of your life...If you want to enjoy life as it was meant to be enjoyed...If you want to be free from the prison that is the 9 to 5 world...If you want to take control instead of being controlled...YOU have to make it happen!

Start making it happen today.

In this book, I will show you how now by taking control of your health.

I promised you that I would show you how to get rid of unsightly cellulite in 10 days and I will deliver the "Cause and Cure" in Chapter 1

"The human mind will first seek to alleviate pain before it seeks pleasure"

The Clown

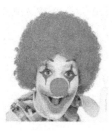

In New York City, on a bright spring day, a man dodges the crowds of pedestrians as he makes his way to a downtown Manhattan skyscraper.

Anyone who would look would see the man was burdened; his hunched shoulders, the look of sadness in his face and eyes, betrayed the man's inner gloom.

The man soon arrives at his destination, an appointment made months in advance, with one of New York's leading psychiatrists.

The man is ushered into the doctor's plush office, and sits heavily in the offered chair.

The doctor asks in a quiet manner, "What seems to be the problem?"

The man hesitates at first, and then finds his voice. He clears his throat and almost whispers, "I really don't know, doctor. I haven't smiled in years. I have no joy in my life. And worst of all, I have no idea why?"

The doctor nods his head, in understanding, and then proceeds to administer a comprehensive battery of tests, beginning with a physical, to determine the cause of the man's problem.

Afterwards, in a private session, the doctor counsels, "I find nothing wrong with you, sir," he begins with a sigh, "but I want you to try something. There is a circus in town this week. They say it is the finest circus in the world. There is a clown with this circus with a reputation of making everyone laugh. I want you to go and see this clown. Possibly, he can restore your joy."

The man looks up from wringing his hands. And with tears in his eyes, he stares at the doctor. Almost in a choking voice the man says, "Doctor, I am that clown!"

On the outside, the man was the epitome of joy... a clown, but on the inside, he was a barren and lonely man.

How many people do you know do the same thing?

It is human nature to project what you want the world to see *(we call this reputation or a facade),* and behind closed doors, the real you comes out *(we call this character).* Remember, a facade is just a mask!

We are what we are in the dark; all the rest is reputation. What God looks at is what we are in the dark-the imaginations of our minds; the thoughts of our heart; the habits of our bodies, these are the things that mark us in God's sight. - Oswald Chambers –

Nutrition and fitness represent one of the largest industries on the net today.

But with all the pertinent information and products available, the only thing they can do and do well is increase the quality of your life rather than the quantity of your life.

Since it is true our days are numbered, it makes sense that these days should be filled with meaning, and a peaceful existence designed to maximize the "quality" of life.

But another human trait has a way of consistently rearing its ugly head: "People are more interested in relief versus cure!"

As long as there is no pain and they look good, people seem content to operate and live their lives within this facade.

This too is wrong and pardon my pun but it is also "dead' wrong!

Always go for QUALITY! The quantity of your life will take care of itself.

Chapter 1 – The Cause and Cure of Cellulite

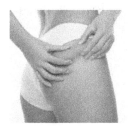

CELLULITE is the scourge of women's thighs and the bane of the female swimsuit industry that causes clothing executives to place their head in their hands and speak in tongues.

Without a doubt the most often asked question of the beauty industry today is, **"How do I get rid of cellulite?"** To begin to answer the question, let's define what cellulite is.

Cellulite is an accumulation of fat globules trapped between the muscle and the skin. If allowed to go unchecked, the fat globules may increase in size and compaction and the result: a quasi-armor plating of fat that robs women of their self-esteem and causes untold misery to millions of American women.

Now that you know what cellulite is, let's define what it IS NOT:

 Cellulite IS NOT related to excess body fat.

 Cellulite IS NOT related to the ingestion of fat in our diets. ELIMINATING DIETARY FAT DOES NOTHING TO CONTROL CELLULITE. Thin women have it as well as obese women.

 Cellulite IS NOT treated by strenuous aerobic exercise. Marathon runners and female bodybuilders have cellulite.

 Cellulite IS NOT caused by fluid trapped in the tissues.

 Cellulite IS NOT eliminated by vigorous massage.

 Cellulite is NOT eliminated by eating high fiber diets and/or diuretic foods (cucumbers, celery, and grapefruit).

Although cellulite most often appears on a woman's upper rear thighs, it can appear elsewhere. It is also now known that cellulite does have a hereditary nature. Cellulite can and does appear on men but it appears less because men have thicker skin. In fact, women have 20% thinner skin than men but have a whopping 50% more body fat.

We also know that a high carbohydrate diet does increase cellulite build-up by increasing the Advanced Glycosycation end-products (AGEs) in the body. These AGEs cross link with proteins and act like little magnets. It is this opposite polarity magnetic effect that causes the hill-and-valley ripple look of cellulite. AGES are known to build-up and cause problems with arteries and DNA.

WHAT IS THE CAUSE OF CELLULITE?

Answer: Cellulite's main cause is the lack of essential fatty acids in your diet.

Everyone is looking for a magic pill to do away with health, nutrition and beauty problems. Magic pills don't exist but in the case of cellulite they do! Yep, to get rid of cellulite quickly and easily go to the store and buy a good Omega 3 formulation or simple flaxseed oil in capsules. A woman should take 4/day of 1000 mgs. Why? All female hormones are manufactured by EFAs. Ladies, are you having hormone problems in menopause or pre-menopause? Go and start taking EFAs. EFAs occur in fish oils, flaxseed oil and as Omega 3 products.

Let's discuss cellulite's annoying hill-and-valley structure. Most of our diets consist of highly processed oils and fats. From these processed oils and fats come Transfatty Acids (TFAs). These TFAs have replaced the necessary and needed essential fatty acids (EFAs) which are body thrives on but of which we obtain very little of in our diets because of the highly processed foods that we consume. Furthermore, these TFAs are not as flexible within the cell wall as the EFAs that they have replaced. Their rigidity interferes with the natural cell flexibility. The lack of cell flexibility magnifies the hill-and-valley effect.

Cellulite is an EFA deficiency indicator.

By understanding the human body, one will see that many problems relate to nutrition. Women especially have different dietary needs than a man. Without a proper diet, women can develop very serious problems.

There are some skeletal differences worth mentioning here. A woman's spine is shorter than a man's spine by about an inch. This is because of childbearing. Also, a woman's pelvis is wider than a man's pelvis and is the reason for the "wiggle" in a woman's walk. It is these two skeletal differences that cause a woman to accumulate fat on her thighs, especially her rear thighs since it is the least problematic area for the body to deposit fat.

A bipedal (two legged) animal has the ability to stand upright by a unique sense of balance found in our inner ear. If the skeleton is misaligned, due to trauma or childbirth, the body will adjust for balance by placing fat in problem areas. In a woman, the adjustment usually occurs in the thighs. Men, being much larger and taller than a woman and consequently having a higher center of gravity, have the adjustment usually centered in the gut area.

Treatment of unsightly cellulite is relatively easy by using the following protocol.

Please Note: The information provided below is for educational purposes only and is not recommended as a means of diagnosing or treating a physical or mental illness or condition. All matters concerning physical or mental health should be supervised by a health practitioner. Although this regimen utilizes only natural supplements, we recommend you notify your health practitioner prior to beginning any new diet regimen.

This Lifestyles Regimen Program involves the following supplements:

Natural Organic Oils (1,000 mgs gel caps recommended) made from a variety of natural oils such as flaxseed, sesame, sunflower, etc. containing:

- Alpha-Linolenic Acid/Omega-3

- Linoleic Acid/Omega-6

- Oleic Acid/Omega-9

Any health food store carries flaxseed oil gel caps; a fair price for 200-count is approximately $15-$16.00. Make sure, by reading the label on the bottle that it is 1,000 mgs, that it contains the three above Omega 3, 6, 9 ingredients. Also, keep the open bottle refrigerated.

Directions: take 3-capsules in the morning 30-minutes before eating and 3-capsules in the evening 30-minutes before eating.

Comprehensive Mineral Supplement (amino acid chelated) containing the following nine essential minerals: boron, iron, magnesium, zinc, selenium, copper, manganese, chromium, potassium, as well as containing the following key ingredients: molybdenum, l-glutamic acid, MSM (methylsulfonylmethane), horsetail extract, sulfer, vanadium, phosphorus, and calcium. Make sure the mineral supplement is amino acid chelated!!! If it is not, you are wasting your money. Furthermore, make sure it contains the above nine essential minerals. The word "essential" means that they are not obtained in your diet and are needed as a supplement.

Directions: Take two (2) tablets daily.

Detoxification Tea containing the following certified organic ingredients: burdock root, sheep sorrel herb, slippery elm bark, watercress herb, Turkish rhubarb root, blessed thistle herb, and red clover blossom. If possible use an Esiac formulation, which is of superior quality. Also, this is the dry formula that you make yourself and is a very good value.

Directions: Follow manufacturer's instructions to make tea as well as dosage amount.

HGH Supplement: an amino acid based precursor that causes the pituitary gland to secrete more human growth hormone.

- Limit ingestion of carbohydrates to 20% of a total dietary intake of 2,000 calories/day. 1 gram of carbs =1tsp. of sugar = 5 calories.

- Light exercise (anaerobic is preferred) is recommended.

Chapter 2 - Toxins and Toxaemia

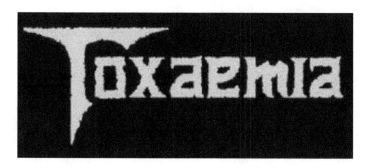

The human body is finely designed to stay in balance (homeostasis) in terms of tissue building up (called anabolism), and tissue breaking down (called catabolism).

An excess of one over the other, is called a metabolic imbalance. Toxaemia (the buildup of toxins in the body), first occurs as a process of metabolism.

Old cells are constantly being replaced by new cells. In fact three hundred billion or more old cells are called toxic, and must be removed, as soon as possible, by the immune system, through one of four channels of elimination: bowels, bladder, lungs, and skin...and sometimes hurling (LOL).

The problem of Toxaemia first occurs when your body is not eliminating toxics at the same rate the toxics are being reproduced.

The second way Toxaemia occurs is from the by-products of foods that are not properly digested.

The major portions of the foods we eat are processed. Because most of our food has been altered from its original state and we are not biologically adapted to deal with this altered food, the by-products of the incomplete digestion form a certain amount of residue, which builds up in the body.

This residue is also called Toxic. Regarding your body weight, common sense will tell you that if more of this toxic weight is built up, rather than eliminated, then obesity will occur.

TOXAEMIA IS THE NUMBER 1 CAUSE OF OBESITY AND NOT A HIGH CALORIE DIET!!!

An excess of body fat holds the toxic wastes and attempts to keep the toxins away from the organs of the body.

Toxins are acidic by nature, hence the body retains water to dilute and neutralize the acids in the toxins, adding even more weight and bloatedness.

If the problem goes unchecked, the ultimate result is not only obesity, but also general discomfort, lethargy and a DISRUPTION OF THE ENERGY FLOW OF THE BODY!

In fact, a good deal of the body's finite energy supply is used to eliminate the toxins in the body.

Cleansing of the system frees up energy.

The following problems occur directly because of Toxaemia:

- Cellulite
- irritable bowel syndrome
- arthritis
- swollen ankles/joints
- bad breath
- slow metabolism (increase in weight)
- ulcers
- digestive problems
- migraines
- bad skin
- weak hair and nails
- low immune system
- and kidney problems

<u>Something to think about…</u>

The concept of total optimum health is not new. This term has been bantered about the healthcare field for years.

What is unique is my belief that total optimum health is only achieved when the needs of the body, mind, soul, and spirit, as they interrelate with one another, are met or exceeded.

In other words, the mind affects the body and the body affects the mind!

There is a common belief among leading social scientists that intellect and emotion never meet. In other words, they are mutually exclusive, and never interrelate with each other in our decision-making processes.

Can this be true?

Let me give an example, and then you can decide. When a person sees a baby crying, the action required to pick-up that baby (intellect), has no bearing whatsoever on the need to pick-up that baby (emotion).

In other words, what is required to raise that baby off the floor against the law of gravity has nothing to do with the desire to hold the baby and give it love and a nurturing environment.

Yes, a physical action is quite different from a nurturing action but the point I am making is that they are both ACTIONS; hence, they are interrelated.

Why is this so important? By understanding the body's relationships, a person can acquire a better quality of life. No science can extend your life, but science can and does offer a better quality of life.

My beliefs regarding health goes against the grain of accepted health field thought.

Contrary to popular belief, most people believe that systematic science puts forth a theory and when this theory is proven then it becomes a law of science.

Einstein put for the theory of relativity in 1903 (e=mc2) and it became the Law of Relativity in 1933 not because anybody proved it. This IS NOT what systemic science does at all! A theory becomes a law if we CANNOT DISPROVE THE THEORY WRONG.
This is called "falsification" and this is how systematic science operates. What you are about to read will be an adventure in thought and practice.

The health world has been telling you for decades to limit your protein and fat intake, and to eat a high-carbohydrate diet.

It is my contention that this high carbohydrate/low fat diet is causing major problems with the health and well being of many Americans.

The incidence of heart disease, diabetes, and cancer are on the rise. So what has caused these problems?

This book will discuss these topics plus much more. Later in the book, we will also discuss the latest in food and health technology…the cutting edge of nutritional research.

We will also discuss the need for supplements.

Do you really need to take all those pills?

Walking into a health store can be a mind-boggling experience. Even most professional health people are hard pressed to tell you how to choose a good supplement.

Also, I want you to pay extra close attention to the chapters dealing with HGH and the Glycemic Food Index.

These are very important chapters, on weight maintenance and body science.

For you ladies, we have included some interesting reports on problems that affect the female body.

In my book "Applied Mind Science," I delve into how the mind affects the body not only in regards to health but also in the total quality of life.

I strongly recommend you read this book! It is well worth the effort and cost. http://store.payloadz.com/go?id=781948 .

Chapter 3 - The sciences and how they interrelate

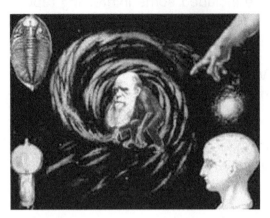

Let's begin by laying down a solid foundation just to keep things in perspective. As previously said, every human being is made up of mind, body, soul, and spirit. The health of a human being centers on all four of these characteristics.

A physical disease will affect mental health, and a mental disease will affect physical health.

It is important to understand that all medical science and practices come from a religious foundation. From the 5th century B. C. up until the mid-1800s, all medicine was practiced based on humoralistic beliefs and techniques.

This practice is attributed to the Greek physician, Hippocrates, but holds a significant resemblance to, the ancient Hindu system called the, "Ayurvedic" system. Humors are the fluids in the human body.

This was the reason a person was "bled," and leeches employed, to remove excess fluids. Once this quackery was debunked, western medicine turned to allopathic practice, or "Allopathy."

Allopathy is a method of treating disease with remedies that produce effects different (dissimilar) from those caused by the disease itself.

Allopathy is the system of medicine practiced today by medical doctors (M.D.s) and relies solely on scientific experimentation.

Allopathy differs from naturopathy; insofar, as the former practices curative medicine, and the latter practices preventative medicine.

Allopathic medicine uses medications and surgery. Naturopathic physicians employ, natural, or alternative methods.

Homeopathy is a system of medicine, or method of treating disease, with remedies that produce effects similar to those caused by the disease itself.

Osteopathy and Chiropractic systems are methods using manipulation of the skeleton, to cure problematic parts of the body.

None of the methods used today, regard the "mind" as influencing the healing process. This is very sad.

Psychology was born in the mid-1800s too. It used to be called philosophy but the desire to make it a "science' overcame the logic of what it truly is and today it operates under a blanket of respectability that is unwarranted.

Remember, systematic science first proposes a theory and when it cannot be disproved (falsification) the theory then becomes a law.

All of psychology is based on the mechanism of the mind: belief systems + thought = behavior/conduct.

Then in 1957, a noted psychologist name Leon Festinger proposed the theory of "cognitive dissonance," which states that actions are inconsistent with beliefs.

This one theory completely contradicts all of psychology!

In psychology's almost 150 years of existence, not one theory has ever been proven or disproven. THERE ARE NO LAWS OF PSYCHOLOGY…not one!

None of psychology's methods used today regard the "mind" as influencing the healing process.

To better understand, the human being, as it relates to others as well as its environment, I need you to thoroughly understand the concept that the "Complete Person" is made up of mind, body, soul, and spirit.

Physiologically speaking, the body operates around the central nervous system; made up of two sub-systems called the somatic nervous system (this is the system that gives you volitional control of your muscles and skeletal movements) and the autonomic nervous system (this is the system, which regulates our glands and correlates with our emotions).

The central nervous system includes the brain, and spinal cord. The autonomic nervous system tells the brain, which stimuli have been received; the brain responds based upon how it has been programmed.

Since an individual is the sum total of his/her experiences, the brain is programmed based on these experiences, as well as perceived experience.

The brain IS NOT the mind! The mind resides in the brain but they are two separate and distinct entities. The best way to describe all of the "parts," using computer terminology, is the autonomic nervous system is the software, the brain is the hardware, and the mind is the hard drive.

You must never forget the "Complete Person" concept, as you attempt to practice proper health protocols. E

very book has a system, a diet, a proven way to lose weight...the claims touted are amazing.

DON'T BELIEVE ANY OF IT!

- If you have a strong desire to be healthy, simply eat good wholesome food; stay away from processed food and adulterated fats.

- Eat natural things like nuts, fruits, and vegetables.

- Remember, too: eat in moderation and only when you are hungry. BALANCE is what you should seek!

- As for supplements, they are not food. They are meant to supplement a diet.

To begin to understand your body, you must first understand the relationships your body employs, as it strives for optimum health.

As a behavioral scientist trained in both secular and non-secular protocols, I have noticed that the secular side of the equation tends to view illness of the body, or the mind, completely separate from the soul and spirit. I referred to this briefly at the end of my book "Addictions" http://www.amazon.com/dp/B006IGHQD4.

Secular psychologists believe that the cause of illness is because of the way we **choose** to think or believe. Using cognitive therapy (having a basis in or reducible to empirical factual knowledge.), they attempt to change a person's behavior and feelings.

But, we now know that illness is cured **not by changing our feelings or behavior,** but **by changing our beliefs and thoughts**.

Does this sound like double-speak to you? One of the things we will discuss is how men/women constantly confuse similar sounding terms, which have very separate and distinct meanings.

In the following, men/women commonly confuse:

 Faith vs. Hope

 Righteousness vs. Goodness

 Freedom vs. Liberty

Rules vs. Ethics

Quality vs. Quantity

Quality of Life vs. Standard of Living

Love vs. Lust

Obligation vs. Legalism

Wealth vs. Money

Want vs. Need

Machismo vs. Manhood

Femininity vs. Womanhood

War vs. Conflict

Well-being vs. Being well

Cause vs. Effect

Relief vs. Cure

Rationalization vs. Right

Promise vs. Oath (Vow)

Discipline vs. Punishment

Taste vs. Substance

Pain vs. Suffering

Self-Control vs. Willpower

Can you honestly tell me the difference between liberty and freedom? Cause and effect, is one example of this problem. Using my statement above, beliefs (belief systems) and thoughts, CAUSE our behavior and feelings, which are in turn, the effects of both belief and thought.

In order to change your behavior and feelings, you must first change the cause; which are your belief systems. You need to reread this paragraph again slowly, because it is very important.

Belief Systems evoke thoughts, which evoke actions, which equal behavior and feelings.

Many people have mental illnesses, which manifests itself in psychosomatic (self-caused) symptoms of depression, anxiety, chronic fatigue, drug addiction, insomnia, ulcers etc.

The mind truly does affect the body!

Think of someone who has wronged you in the past, and see how your body responds. You become anxious and stressed. You begin to think of revenge, as your heart races, and your ears pound. Adrenaline begins to course through your body. You cannot separate the two entities (body and mind always interact), even though there are some occult religions that claim to free you from your body by meditation and visualization.

In the above example, you react the way you do based on how your mind has been programmed. This is your character. A child reared in a family, which uses violence to solve problems, uses violence in its own life, to solve problems, because this is how the child was programmed.

A lifestyle is made up of various habits. All people respond, to various stimuli, based on how they are trained. Over the years, people have learned to react to certain situations with a predictable behavioral pattern.

Habits through practice turn into behavior - both good and bad. Like I said, not all habits are good habits either. A person suffers from his/her own personal problems, like you, and the stress and anxiety his/her choices bring.

Wrongful choices evoke stress and anxiety. This is important to understand completely. Wrongful choices evoke suffering. This suffering takes the form of anxiety, stress, and the list of other psychosomatic ailments I previously listed.

Here is a direct quote from one of my associates, psychologist Hobart Mowrer, that I think you will find quite interesting:

"Human anxiety is a result of dammed-up moral force rather than dammed-up libido. As this force seeps out into a man's consciousness (from his subconscious mind), **he experiences it not as guilt about a real fault or sin** (perception) **but as great anxiety. Anxiety is not the result of too little indulgence, but of too much, not of over-restraint and inhibition, but of irresponsibility, guilt, and immaturity. Above all, the eternal accomplishment of untold past generations, as imbedded in the conscience of modern men and women, is not a stupid, malevolent, archaic incubus** (evil spirit), **but a challenge and guide for the individual, in his quest for self-fulfillment and harmonious integration."**

Freud regarded anxiety as foreign, unfriendly, and destructive. However, Mowrer believes that conscience, and the anxiety it produces, can be transformed into guilt and moral fear, for which unhappy man can make some realistic adjustment. Mowrer's prescription: A changed attitude (belief system) toward social authority and its internal representative anxiety. We will also talk more about authority in just a little while.

"If a man's attitude is not changed, he will continue to seek relief from anxiety in such futile devices as tobacco, alcohol, gambling, sexual perversion, and gluttony."

Do you get it? Some of the things you do are caused by stress and anxiety, which have been caused by wrongful choices. Smoking, over-eating, drinking, and gambling, are just a few examples of the manifested behavior caused by stress and anxiety, which in turn, are caused by wrongful choices.

These types of manifested behaviors act as a relief valve and defense mechanism. It follows that since wrongful choices are the true culprit to a life of bondage, to the effects of wrongful choices, then we need to learn how to develop correct choices.

Let me take it one step further. People do not appear to see the difference between the matter part of an organism and the life part, which animates it. They seem to think that the organism itself is life. We all seem to suffer a similar problem of understanding.

To put it in perspective, people do not appear to see the difference between their outward habits and the inward part that animates it. It is not their outward appearance that defines their habits but their inward experiences and anxieties, and this is where their habits are born.

In other words, life is not your physical body. Life is what animates the body. Life is your spirit, but the soul of man has usurped the spirit's position and psychology is now forced to define "how" we live our lives based on the animating force of the soul instead of the spirit.

To summarize, the body contains the brain, which contains the mind, which contains the conscious and subconscious parts of the mind. The subconscious mind is made up of the desires, emotions and will or what I refer to as "DEW". This is where we get our feelings, attitudes, sentiments and opinions. This is where our dreams are born and failures grieved. This is the place where intricate processes are put into motion and life's decisions are contemplated.

Here we find the conflicting emotions of love/hate, like/dislike, and attraction/repulsion. Here is our daily existence. It is the pollution of the subconscious mind that causes our problems. All manifested behavior stems from the subconscious mind! The soul of man is a term to describe this subconscious aspect of man.

The ancient Hebrews defined the soul in two ways. They called the souls of animals "nefesh," which were souls that did not share the eternality nature of God, and the soul of man was called "neshama," which did share the eternality of God.

All animals possess souls (science uses the term "breath" to describe the physical manifestation of the soul); it is our spirits, which makes us different.

The mind is very important because this is the playground of poor choices. It is in the mind where all thought is first contemplated and it is in the mind where all action begins.

"On the inside, we are defined by what we lack, on the outside, what defines us is what we have."

What we lack on the inside is Truth and what we have on the outside is what the world uses to evaluate our success.

Now getting back to the mind, we know that our minds can be used against us. Everyone has heard of brainwashing, mind-control, magic, hypnosis, etc. To live in the mind, we live as "consuming entities." We desire to take and not give back. Look around you, the world always wants more. We even call ourselves "consumers".

The products we consume are offered up in the most appealing advertisements. They are "beautiful" and we want them. In olden times, our eyes were never bigger than our pocketbook. We didn't have credit cards back then. Today, we can consume on credit and this has led many into a life of financial subjugation.

"If you live as a consuming entity, you will always lose."

In other words, to get, you must give-you must sacrifice! Have you ever wondered why you have so many anxieties, phobias, worries and fears?

Remember what I taught you above. The reality of this world is evil. So what is reality? I will tell you. This is reality:

"Life without war is impossible either in nature or in grace. The basis of physical, mental, moral and spiritual life is antagonism. Health is the balance between physical life and external nature, and it is maintained only by sufficient vitality on the inside against things on the outside.

Everything outside my physical life is designed to put me to death.

Things, which keep me going when I am alive, disintegrate

me when I am dead. If I have enough fighting power, I produce the balance of health. The same is true of mental life. If I want to maintain a vigorous mental life, I have to fight, and in that way the mental balance called thought is produced. Morally it is the same. Everything that does not partake of the nature of virtue is the enemy of virtue in me, and it depends on what moral caliber I have whether I overcome and produce virtue (GOOD CHARACTER). Immediately I fight, I am moral in that particular. No man is virtuous because he cannot help it; virtue (character) is acquired.

Chapter 4 - Do You Really Need All Those Supplements?

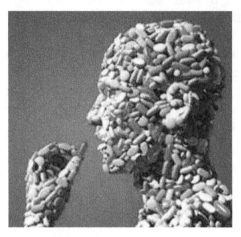

In answering a question as complicated and important as this one, we must look to scientific fact rather than the host of opinions that bombard the American consumer. One fact is this: the optimum daily amounts of vitamins and minerals are far larger than the amounts that can be obtained in food. This is because of present day farming techniques and an increase in the amount of processed food Americans ingest daily. The quality has decreased and Americans have increased the quantity of consumption. Poor food and poor eating habits require us to use supplements.

Choosing a Responsibly Made Vitamin

Vitamins either enable biochemical reactions in the body to take place more effectively, or they prevent specific substances from interfering with the biochemical reactions.

Why do I need to take vitamins?

If our soil was not depleted and we did not use pesticides and herbicides on our crops, which greatly reduce the bioavailability of the nutrients to be metabolized, and we ate fruits and vegetables within 6-days of harvesting, and we didn't heat process our food, and add preservatives to them-we wouldn't need to take vitamins.

What should I look for in a vitamin?

Consumers need to be well informed when making the decision to ingest any substance. In considering a supplement, the guidelines for determining if a supplement is responsibly made should include: Heat Processing and Tableting, Iron -Why it should NOT be present, Vitamin-C, Vitamin-D, Beta Carotene, B-Complexes, Chelation and Minerals, Timed-Released, and Synergists.

Heat Processing and Tableting

Look for a supplement that is not heat processed.

Tablets are heat processed and capsules are not. Capsules cost the manufacturer more, so most manufacturers tend to use the tableting method. Capsules or pure powders deliver the highest potency. Also, fillers and binders are used to make a tablet hold together, and these binders may cause allergic reactions in some people. Many people think they are allergic to vitamins when they are really only allergic to the binder or filler. Also, tableting may cause extrusion of oil-soluble vitamins from the formulation. For example, a tablet press compresses at 5000 psi which can release beadleted oil-soluble Vitamin A from the protective coat. The Vitamin A then degrades rapidly.

Iron – Why it Should NOT be Present

Look for a complete vitamin/mineral supplement that does not contain iron.

Studies have shown that "increased body iron stores are associated with an increase risk of cancer": New England Journal of Medicine. This does not refer to iron found in food or the iron found in protein powders, but to supplemental iron. Also, studies indicate that two-in-four hundred Caucasians have Hemochromatosis; an inherited disorder that causes iron overload and the symptoms can be quite severe. Iron deficiencies in males are rare. Some women do have iron deficiencies in which case an increase in dietary intake of iron rich foods may eliminate the problem. If dietary readjustment does not alleviate the deficiency, an iron supplement may be taken once or twice a week until serum iron levels reach the normal range.

Vitamin-C

The data on Vitamin-C is so extensive that it is unnecessary to validate its value. I would not take more than 500 mgs of Vitamin-C per day.

Megadoses are not advisable

(Are we really meant to consume 20-30 oranges a day? Does this make sense to you?). Megadoses of Vitamin-C depress sperm motility and decreases fertility. It also blunts the beneficial effects of chemotherapy treatment for breast cancer. Cancer cells have numerous receptors for Vitamin-C making it act as a growth tonic for cancer cells. Also, its own synergist, the bioflavonoids, should always accompany Vitamin-C. Vitamin-C does not occur in nature without its sisters, rutin and hesperidin-both bioflavonoids, and any well-made vitamin should mimic nature as closely as possible. Note: Smoking depletes almost 50% of the vitamin-C in the body.

Vitamin-D

Vitamin-D is a vitamin, which acts like a hormone and is the only vitamin the human body can manufacture. In its absence, calcium and phosphorus become immobile and leeching of these two minerals becomes inevitable. In addition, as we age, our ability to synthesize Vitamin-D slows to one-half. Though we need Vitamin-D, it is potentially very toxic, so a safe supplement will not contain large amounts of Vitamin-D. We do not recommend taking a Vitamin-D supplement.

If your body is getting the proper amount of essential fatty acids (Omega 3, 6, 9 oils) your body will make a sufficient amount of Vitamin-D.

Most of the Vitamin-D utilized in the body comes from sunlight interacting with the essential fatty acids in the skin. Therefore, supplemental Vitamin-D without the benefit of sunlight is insufficient for total health. Sun exposure (with sunscreen) should include 20-minutes of summer sun exposure and 40-minutes of winter sun exposure. Be advised that an excessive amount of Vitamin-D causes a magnesium deficiency in the body. Furthermore, megadoses of Vitamin-D irritate the lining of blood vessels and are one of the causes of atherosclerosis.

Beta Carotene

Beta Carotene (Pro-Vitamin A or plant derived Vitamin A) is a natural substance found in fruits and vegetables, which, once inside the body, converts to Vitamin A. Vitamin A is crucial in normal cellular control. Since the body must get Vitamin A from outside sources, when the body does not receive an adequate supply of Vitamin A, cell function becomes abnormal, and cell maturation does not take place. Cells deprived of Vitamin A dedifferentiate, and enter a state paralleling cancerous cells. Stress (including both colds and flu) can deplete up to 60% of the Vitamin A in the body. At St. Luke's Medical Center in Chicago, an important study involving beta-carotene and lung cancer was conducted. It involved 2,107 workers at the Western Electric Company in Chicago. Thirty-Three (33) of the men developed lung cancer, all related to cigarette smoking. The rate of cancer was lowest in those people consuming the highest amounts of beta-carotene foods and the highest in the group consuming the least amounts of beta-carotene foods. The actual ratio turned out to be an 8-to-1 difference in risk between the lowest and highest groups. Beta Carotene can actually negate gene mutation, which occurs when the body is exposed to environmental toxins such as cigarette smoke. The incidence of lung cancer in smokers (2 packs a day for 30-years) who consumed diets high in beta-carotene was similar to the incidence of lung cancer in non-smokers. This is phenomenal data evidencing the powerful anti-carcinogenic properties of beta-carotene. Unused Vitamin A is stored in the liver and can be toxic when taken for extended periods at high doses, where as beta-carotene is considered nontoxic at very high doses. A combination of beta-carotene and Vitamin A (in moderate doses) in a supplement is preferable.

B-Complexes

The B-Vitamins include: B-1 (Thiamin), B-2 (Riboflavin), B-5 (pantothenic acid), B-6 (pyridoxine), B-12 (Cobalamin), PABA (para-aminobenzoic acid), folate (folic acid), inositol, biotin and choline.

Because of modern food processing, it is extremely difficult to obtain even the minimum amount of B-Complexes from our food alone.

Current labeling shows the amount of nutrients found in a food before processing, not after. Flour, for example, loses 82% of its B-vitamins in processing, and spaghetti 64%. Even cracked wheat bread has lost 38% of its B-vitamins. A deficiency of just one of the B-vitamins, thiamin causes extreme mood swings due to lack of availability of serotonin, a brain chemical which help regulate emotions. Patients complaining of lethargy, personality changes, and sleep disturbances, lack of appetite, diarrhea, and fevers of unknown origin were studied. These symptoms "would represent a trap for the unwary physician since he would be unable to find any objective physical sign other than variations of normal, which would be easily classed as the effects of a chronic state of anxiety" (American Journal of Clinical Nutrition). When supplemental Thiamin was given, all patients in the study reported a marked symptomatic improvement or a complete loss of all symptoms.

Ingestion of coffee, either regular or decaffeinated, severely depletes Thiamin. Thiamin isn't alone in its ability to affect moods. Niacin depletion causes severe reactions in humans. "If all the niacin were removed from our food, everyone wood be psychotic in one year," (Abram Hoffer, MD and psychiatrist). B-vitamins are also catalysts in the burning of carbohydrates and in glucose tolerance. B-vitamins are water-soluble (Oil-soluble vitamins are A, D, E, and K) so taking them in the morning with breakfast and again with lunch will help insure high energy throughout the day. There are many good quality B-complex supplements for women available in health stores. Be sure to read the labels and understand what you are ingesting. Niacin can cause "flushing" in doses over 30-50mgs, so you may wish to take niacin separately and use a supplement with the "non-flushing" form of niacin, "niacinamide". Niacinamide lacks the beneficial vasodialating effects found in niacin, but "flushing" frightens those who do not understand that flushing is beneficial and is often replaced by niacinamide for that reason.

Chelation and Minerals

Without the proper minerals, vitamins cannot be fully utilized.

Minerals are the building blocks for body tissue and other body structures. Minerals enable enzymes and hormones, which regulate the metabolism. Also, minerals maximize the efficiency of healthy essential oils containing the all-important essential fatty acids. Minerals are inorganic and are co-enzymes. Our bodies cannot use raw minerals when taken in their inorganic form because they cannot be digested or used. Plants transform minerals from the soil into an organic form that humans can use by eating vegetables as well as eating animals that have eaten plants and have the minerals present in their meat. The minerals in a supplement should be chelated (bound or "hooked up") to another substance such as an amino acid to promote better bioavailability. Most mineral supplements commonly described as "chelated" have an organic molecule like a citrate or gluconate chemically tied to the mineral, which has a very low bioavailability. Since the intestinal wall readily absorbs proteins, avoid the following so-called chelating agents that are not protein based: citrates, sulfates, gluconates, phosphates, etc.). Chelated minerals are less irritating to the gastrointestinal tract compared to some of the salts of these minerals. We waste money on supplements the body cannot use effectively. For example: By swallowing a 200mg pill of calcium less than 14% is used by the body which translates into 28% bio-availability. Take a 500mg pill of calcium and the body uses almost 70%. How effectively a nutritional supplement is absorbed is far more important than how much is taken. For example: the calcium absorption rate for milk is 30%. For ideal mineral absorption, the ration of minerals to amino acid bonding must be in the ratio between 1-unit of mineral to 3-units of amino acid; the weight of the amino acids in the mineral chelate must be very small (150 Daltons), the total molecular weight must be less than 800 Daltons, and the chelate must not ionize in the digestive system. Digestion quickly separates the commonly used chelating mineral salts or complexes from any mixed-in protein. We want the mineral-protein combination to remain free of positive or negative ions. Otherwise, the mineral will bond with something else and may not be utilized. Note: It is for this reason we suggest that you do not use "Colloidal Minerals!

A mineral plays three roles in the human body:

☆ It supports the energy conversion process

☆ It aids in the growth and maintenance of the body's tissues

☆ They assist in the regulation of all bodily processes.

Contrary to popular belief, chelation does not insure absorption of minerals, as this is best achieved by taking mineral supplements with food containing minerals.

The ingestion of fresh food is always the best way to achieve maximum nutrient intake. Individual biochemistry, including enzymatic functions, will generally determine a person's ability to effectively process minerals. However, minerals tied to salts have little bioavailability compared to amino acid chelation.

There are 17 minerals, which humans need. The following nine minerals (out of the seventeen) are essential; insofar, as they are not found in our food supply: boron, iron, magnesium, zinc, selenium, copper, manganese, chromium, and potassium. A good mineral supplement should contain the above nine essential minerals, plus calcium, and phosphorus.

If the supplement lists all of the minerals in equal doses, opt for another choice, as minerals do not occur in nature in equal amounts. Do not rely on a supplement to supply you with all the minerals you need.

Eat fresh vegetables and fruit, beans, fish, turkey and chicken and take a well-formulated vitamin/mineral supplement with fresh food.

Timed-Released

It is better not to use timed-released vitamins.

There are exceptions, of course, but they are rare. When it comes to absorption, timed-released nutrients are inferior. Timed-released vitamins are a nice concept, but research shows conclusively that with a timed-released vitamin, the percent of dosage absorbed is low compared to that of a regular non timed-released vitamin. This is especially true of Vitamin-C.

Synergists

Certain vitamins taken without their synergistic sisters are better off not taken at all.

No one nutrient occurs in nature all by itself. When Vitamin-C is present in fruit, its sister, the bioflavonoids, always accompanies it. This is extremely important! Minerals occur in nature in certain ratios to each other and they work synergistically, as do the B-vitamins. A good example is cystine. Do not take supplemental cystine without taking at least 3-times as much Vitamin-C as cystine. Taking large amounts of cystine without Vitamin-C can cause cystine stones in the kidneys and urinary bladder. Well made vitamin and mineral supplements are an excellent adjunct to food, but be an informed and aware consumer when choosing your supplements. As you read this book, you will be given valuable information, which is necessary to live a good quality of life. Remember balance and moderation is important too.

Did you know?

   Milk is the probable leading cause of Heart Disease?

   May lead to an increased risk of breast cancer?

   The powerful growth hormones in milk increase the rate

of cancer growth.

 The body does not adequately absorb calcium in milk.

 Milk consumption is the probable cause of osteoporosis.

Chapter 5 - Essential Fatty Acids

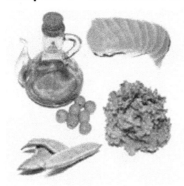

When people say the word "FAT" they immediately think of a food that could add unsightly pounds to their waistline, causing them to gain unnecessary weight. This is just plain wrong! There are "good" fats and "bad" fats and the beneficial ones can actually help decrease the desire to eat the harmful ones. Fats do many things for the body.

Fats, also known as "lipids", are the body's prime source of energy (not carbs).

They balance the body's chemistry and help with the transportation and absorption of fat-soluble vitamins such as vitamins A, D, E, and K. But their most important function is as a source of the vital nutrients known as essential fatty acids (EFAs). Essential Fatty Acids are vital to our body's need for many functions. They are found in seeds of plants and in oils of cold-water fish. EFAs are sometimes referred to as Vitamin F. Since our bodies cannot make EFAs, they must be supplied by our diet. Here is a list of the vital functions EFAs accomplish in our bodies:

   Lowers triglyceride levels.

   Helps eradicate plaque from arterial walls.

   Lowers blood pressure.

   Alters the production of leukotrienes, which aggravate inflammation in the body. This is good news to those suffering from arthritis, lupus, psoriasis and other inflammation-related ailments.

☆ Helps to construct body membranes working with cholesterol and protein to repair old cell membranes and construct new ones.

☆ Helps to strengthen cell and capillary structures.

☆ Prolongs blood-clotting time.

☆ Helps in the manufacture of hemoglobin, the compound in the blood that provides oxygen to the cells from the lungs.

☆ Assists in the manufacture of cholesterol and also removes excess cholesterol from the blood. Cholesterol has gotten some undeserved press. Cholesterol is a waxy alcohol and is necessary for many vital bodily functions. Interestingly enough, there is no known cholesterol-sensing mechanism in the body. This tells us that an abundance of cholesterol is not a cause for alarm. It is found in the bile, blood, brain tissue, liver, kidneys, adrenal glands, and the myelin sheath of nerve fibers. It helps absorb and transport EFAs and is necessary for the body to synthesize vitamin D. All hormones are made from cholesterol. The body will actually manufacture cholesterol from dietary by-products of proteins, sugars and fats (by cells, glands, the small intestine and the liver) to insure a continuous supply of this important fat. If your diet contains excessive saturated fats, the body will convert them into cholesterol. People who eat high sugar or fat diets may therefore experience elevated cholesterol levels.

☆ Prevents the growth of bacteria and viruses, which will not thrive in the presence of oxygen, by oxygenating cell membranes. Highly unsaturated fatty acids have the ability to hold oxygen and this results in increasing resistance to disease, increased endurance, better metabolic efficiency and energy conversion, plus the balancing of sleep-wake cycles. And for you workout nuts, EFAs also shorten the recovery times for tired muscles.

☆ Assists in the functions of glands and hormones. (Note: EFAs must be present along with vitamins E and B to produce sex and adrenal hormones.)

☆ Nourishes skin, hair and nails. EFAs help to eliminate eczema, psoriasis, dandruff, and help prevent hair loss.

☆ Increases the rate the body burns fat.

☆ Helps maintain the body's temperature.

☆ Assists in the body's production of electrical currents vital for a regular heartbeat.

☆ Acts as a precursor to the production of hormone-like substances called prostaglandins. Prostaglandins are found in almost all body cells and act as catalysts for many physiological processes. They help prevent abnormal blood clotting and nerve inflammation. Prostaglandins also help promote blood circulation by dilating the blood vessels and improve immune system function. The most beneficial type of prostaglandin is called PGE-1, which balances cholesterol and blood pressure levels, and stimulates the body's production of T-lymphocytes, which strengthen the immune capabilities. Each cell keeps tiny amounts of EFAs and produces prostaglandins from them, as they are needed. The name prostaglandins were coined because these substances were originally found in high amounts in the prostate gland. There are 36 different prostaglandins with a wide range of roles in the body.

"Stress, allergies, disease, and a diet high in fried food, increase the body's need for EFAs"

Let's discuss the types of fats.

Saturated Fats

All fats are composed of carbon, hydrogen, and oxygen molecules. The carbon atoms of fatty acids hold together in a chain-like fashion. These carbon atoms can attach hydrogen to them. When each place that can hold a hydrogen atom is filled and there is no room for even one more atom, they are described as "saturated". The longer the chain, the harder the fat will be and hence, the higher its melting point. These types of "long-chain fatty acids" are found in hard fats such as those in red meat, cheese, sour cream, and palm kernel and coconut oils.

Unsaturated Fats:

These fats are called unsaturated because there are at least two adjacent carbon atoms on a chain, which are not attached to hydrogen atoms. When at least two pairs of carbon atoms are empty, it is known as a monounsaturated fatty acid. When two or more sets are empty, then it is referred to as a polyunsaturated fatty acid. Fatty acids are either essential or nonessential. They are essential if the body cannot synthesize them and the only way they can be obtained is through the diet. As far back as the 1930s, researchers discovered that a lack of EFAs in our diets caused poor reproduction, lowered immunity, rough and dry skin, and slow growth

There are basically three essential fatty acids:

1. Linolenic Acid (Alpha-Lenolenic Omega-3.)

The most common forms of Omega-3 are eicosapentaenioic acid (EPA), docisahexaenoic acid (DHA), and alpha-linolenic acid, which come from plants and help create EPA and DHA. Omega-3 is usually derived from fish oils.

Note: Fish Oils containing Omega-3 found in coldwater fish are salmon, bluefish, herring, tuna, and mackerel.

2. Linoleic Acid (Omega-6)

This is the most vital of the EFAs. The other two, linolenic and arachidonic acids can be converted from linoleic acid. It is plant derived and in its most common form, gamma-linolenic acid (GLA) it is known to provide the following benefits:

- Helps facilitate weight loss in overweight persons (but not in people who do not need to lose weight).

- Reduces platelet aggregation (abnormal blood clotting).

- Helps reduce symptoms of depression and schizophrenia.

- Alleviates premenstrual syndrome symptoms.

- May help alcoholics overcome their addiction.

Note: Plants that contain Omega-6 are Black Currant Seed Oil, Borage Oils, Flaxseed Oil, and Evening Primrose

3. Arachidonic Acid

Is unique in that it is abundant in brain cells as well as other cells. To the cell membrane, this acid is critical but elsewhere it may not be so beneficial.

<u>EFA Deficiency Symptoms</u>

A lack of Linoleic Acid can cause adverse symptoms including:

- Acne

- Changes in personality or behavior

- Gallbladder dysfunction

- Slow wound healing

- Cardiovascular problems

- Prostate inflammation

- Thirst due to excessive perspiration

- Arthritis

- ☆ Miscarriage
- ☆ Poor Growth
- ☆ Kidney problems
- ☆ Muscle Tremors
- ☆ Skin disorders
- ☆ Sterility in males

A lack of Linolenic Acid can cause adverse symptoms including:

- ☆ Poor Growth
- ☆ Learning disability
- ☆ Tingling in the extremities
- ☆ Impaired motor coordination
- ☆ Poor Vision

The human body requires forty-five (45) known essential nutrients and it requires linolenic acid (Omega-3) more than any other (at least 6-grams/day). Of the forty-five needed nutrients, 20 are minerals, 15 are vitamins, 8 are amino acids and 2 are fatty acids. Altered fatty acids are called Trans-fatty Acids and are extremely bad for the body. Stay away from deep fried foods. Heated fats, especially of the vegetable kind, may turn into cancer-causing agents by causing free-radical damage to the body. The body CANNOT use trans-fatty acids so they simply collect around fatty tissues and the body's organs. Studies show that EFAs may be helpful for many chronic stubborn conditions. The EFAs' ever growing repertoire of valuable applications includes overcoming diseases such as alcoholism, breast cancer, and cardiovascular disease, strengthening the immune system, helping eliminate yeast infection, reducing symptoms of premenstrual syndrome, minimizing inflammation of rheumatoid arthritis, and assisting in the proper management of weight.

Chapter 6 - Did You Know?

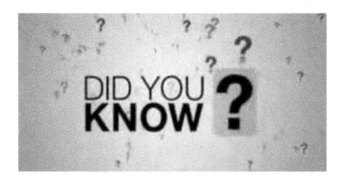

This section offers some very interesting facts that disprove the prevailing health mindset.

 Fat is the body's preferred energy source (not carbs and sugar!). Per unit weight, fats occupy less volume and produce more energy than carbs or protein. One (1) gram of fat produces 2.5 times as much energy as one (1) gram of carbs. We have enough body fat for weeks of survival but only approximately 24-hours of carb reserve.

 Insulin stops fat burning even while exercising.

 Eating fat does not make you fat. Carbs are stored as fat.

 Glucosamine sulfate is not the best thing for joint pain relief because of its effect on inhibiting hepatic glucokinase, the body's glucose sensor.

 Attention Deficit Disorder (ADD) and Attention Deficit Hyperactivity Disorder (ADHD) can be reduced by supplementation of Omega 3 and 6 oils. Lack of EPAs contributes to hyperactivity in kids. Boys are much more affected and males need more EFAs than females.

 Elevated triglyceride levels (bad) persisted throughout the day induced by high carbs, despite the decrease in fat in the diet. High carb diets are associated with increases in both fasting and postprandial (after eating)

triglyceride concentrations.

Substituting carbs for saturated fat leads to higher triglyceride and lower HDL.

The number one health complaint is chronic fatigue.

We consume 160 lbs of sugar per year.

Five (5) grams of carbs equals one (1) teaspoon of sugar. A 12 oz. Can of soda has 35-45 grams of carbs, which equals 7-9 teaspoons of sugar into your bloodstream at one time.

We dump more than 450 teaspoons of sugar into are bloodstreams every week; however our bodies were designed to run on less than 1-teaspoon per week.

1 pound of body fat equals 3500 stored calories.

One 8oz. glass of orange juice has enough sugar in it to provide the energy to run one mile.

The body can manufacture ALL of the carbs it needs from proteins and body fat.

Eating the right kind of fats reduces body fat

Carbs are the worst fuel for achieving peak performance

Carbs stop you from using the fat stored in your own body as the best fuel available.

In 1900 3% died from heart disease. Today, 46% die from heart disease. The jump in heart disease began in the 1930s; the same decade processed cooking oils began widespread usage. A few years later, margarine replaced butter and processed oils virtually eliminated lard. Today, the average American consumes 10 lbs of chemically processed shortening and 20 lbs of margarine each year.

Death from heart disease DECREASES 44% with the use of Omega-3 oils.

If you get food cravings, and frequently run low on

energy; if you need 8-hours or more of sleep; if you have cellulite; if you need three meals each day; if you ever feel intensely hungry and/or stressed out, then you fail the healthy eating test.

- ☆ The cause of plaque build-up in the arteries are tiny cuts or wounds to the arterial wall caused by insulin whereas the body, needing to repair these cuts, places cholesterol as a "scab" eventually leading to a build-up or blockage called plaque.

- ☆ Presumably, the cholesterol in the LDL, coming from the liver to the tissues, is more likely to be deposited at the sites of the arterial wall lesions and cholesterol in the HDL, traveling to the liver, is less likely to contribute to the lesion. Hence LDL cholesterol has the label "bad" and HDL cholesterol has the label "good".

- ☆ The only reason we are eating so many calories is because food processing removes or destroys essential nutrients, triggering the body to signal hunger in hope of getting what it needs.

- ☆ The human gut is proportionately many times longer than that of a strict carnivore. Humans have a weaker stomach acid concentration (10-times weaker than a carnivore). Carnivores need a shorter, more powerful gut to quickly digest raw meat, bone and feathers. Humans are omnivores.

- ☆ Fresh fish has NO smell and tastes buttery. A fishy smell is a sign that the EFAs are going bad.

- ☆ This is something to take into consideration: Virtually all research is conducted on test subjects that are EFA-deficient.

- ☆ The female breast contains a very high proportion of fat cells. Our bodies tend to concentrate and store toxins in fat tissues; hence, we should expect toxins from the air, water and food to build up in a woman's breast tissue, which may cause the increase in breast cancer.

- ☆ Genetic problems are not the cause of obesity. A gene

cannot act by itself; it must combine with other genes to produce a noticeable trait and even then, a gene only presents tendency. They do not dictate actions. Since there is no known genetic cause for obesity, there is no need for medical intervention. Since the problem has a nutritional root, it must be solved by a nutrition-related solution. This is why drug companies need to step back from offering a medical-related solution. Being drugged for a lifetime is not the solution.

 The body has to quickly convert carbs to fat because toxic by-products are formed during the cell's use and breakdown of glucose. If these by-products cannot be used by the body fast enough, they are converted directly to fat and cholesterol to protect us from self-poisoning.

 This is really going to shock you. Studies show that vigorous exercise offers virtually no additional mortality protection over moderate exercise. When your body has the optimal amount of EFAs, your endurance increases and exercise becomes easier.

 A person burns 10-times as much glucose doing anaerobic exercise compared to the same amount of aerobic exercise.

 It would take 10-hours of walking or 5-hours of aerobics to burn 1-pound of body fat.

A person eating 20% carbs/ 80% protein and natural fats after just 10-minutes of aerobics is burning 50% of energy from body fat. After 1-hour it is 65%!

 A typical government recommended diet of 2000 calories/day contains as much as 1200 calories from carbs, which is equivalent to 60-teaspoons of sugar.

 If you are thin and consume large quantities of food without weight gain, beware; this is often the main symptom of the onset of diabetes because the person is not metabolizing much of the food. A glycohemoglobin test will detect diabetes.

- Salt is required for cellular sugar transfer.

- Our brain feeds on glucose and uses two-thirds of the circulating glucose in the bloodstream.

- A typical 180 lb male has 15% body fat or 27 pounds. Twenty-percent (5-7 Pounds) is used structurally throughout the body, so approximately 20 pounds of fat is excess body fat called adipose tissue. A typical 130-pound female has 22% body fat or 29 pounds.

- There is a big difference between thriving and surviving

- Only 1% of your pancreas can be used to make insulin. The other 99% is involved in other various digestive processes. The pancreas is not a muscle like the heart, which works continuously. It is designed to secrete insulin once or twice a day in response to carbohydrates with several hours between secretions. Is it any wonder with the high carb diets that we have virtually worn our pancreas out?

- By taking EFAs 20-30-minutes before meals means you'll desire less food.

- Here's a real shocker: More than two-thirds of all the deaths reported in the United States involves nutrition.

- When you eat natural fat, it goes directly into your lymphatic system-NOT into the bloodstream. A protein must be placed around the fat before it enters the bloodstream. There is no loose fat running around in your bloodstream.

- An average 130-pound female requires a full pound of protein per day for normal body processes. This could be in the form of a high quality whey protein powder but preferably food.

- More than 50% of your body weight is protein. Amino acids are made from protein.

- There are 20 amino acids. The human body can produce

11 of these. That leaves 9, which are called essential amino acids: Histidine, Lysine, Threonine, Isoleucine, methionine, Tryptophan, Leucine, Phenylalanine, and Valine.

Triglycerides are fat made from carbohydrates.

Salt is not bad for you! If you eat too much salt, the body's equilibrium systems go into action and counteract it, i.e. "The Atrial Naturietic Factor" (ANF), which triggers kidneys to dump sodium. Human cells contain almost 1% salt-based nutrients. Stomach acid requires chloride from salt.

For deep-frying use peanut oil or coconut oil. For all other cooking use olive oil. Tropical oils do not raise cholesterol levels.

Brown age spots or "liver" spots are indicative of degeneration in the body. EFAs cause them to become lighter or disappear.

Women taking oral contraceptives and exercising have a significantly higher risk of developing a prethrombic (blood clot) condition.

Here is another shocker: Osteoporosis is not caused by a lack of calcium in the bloodstream. The following are the causes: Lack of physical stress on the bone from inactivity, shortage of protein, lack of vitamin C, postmenopausal lack of estrogen, decrease in growth hormone (HGH) and other hormones inhibiting bone matrix, and Cushings disease (adrenal tumor)

Never use hormone supplements unless prescribed. A tiny bit of hormone causes drastic changes in the body. All hormone production typically decreases with age. Many hormones (and all postaglandins) are made from EFAs.

DHEA is converted in the body into androgens and other steroid hormones.

The definition for appetite is the desire for food; hunger is the need for food.

 The myth of increasing the metabolism to burn more fat wrongly implies that the body is a heat engine when the truth is that it is a chemical engine.

 RDA for fat is 65 grams/day based on a 2000 cal/day diet.

Chapter 7 - The Glycemic Index and HGH

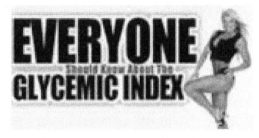

I want to steer you into a new nutritional thought pattern, one that is "contrary" to the accepted "parroted" line that high carbohydrate/low fat and protein diets are what is best for optimum health. If you believe this then you really need to read this report.

Optimum health is achieved when the mind-body-soul are at their peak of efficiency. We achieve the body side of the equation by replacing the essential fatty acids that the high carbohydrate/low fat diets have removed. The American people are addicted to carbohydrates due to the highly processed nature of our food supply.

Optimum health utilizes a mineral supplement that replaces the nine essential minerals that are not found in our food supply. Furthermore, the program calls for a detoxifying tea that removes the accumulation of toxins from the body. As the body releases its excess fat stores, the toxins, which are stored in the adipose (fat) tissues, are released.

Last, our program utilizes a Human Growth Hormone (HGH) precursor formulation and it is this we will now address.

Human Biochemistry, Human Growth Hormone and Positive Nitrogen Balance

Positive nitrogen balance is achieved by having more amino acids going into the body than going out. Excess amino acids are stored as fat unless there is HGH present. The equation looks like this:

Excess amino acids + HGH =Muscle

Excess amino acids - HGH = Stored Fat

To increase the release of HGH by the pituitary gland naturally there must be an increase in physical exercise, an increase in sleep plus the biochemical response to a HGH precursor formulation, which is widely available on the health market today. Release of HGH plus your low carb diet equals: increased lean muscle mass, increased strength, reduced body fat, steady anabolic rate and increased endurance. HGH determines whether dietary protein is converted to fat or muscle. If you want to add lean muscle mass, you will have to exercise, stimulate HGH with an HGH precursor formulation, decrease total carbohydrate consumption to low or moderate glycemic carbs and increase the intake of properly balanced proteins and minerals and fat. Yes I said FAT! Contrary to popular belief, **the body's preferred energy source is not carbohydrates. It is FAT!**

What is the difference between high and low glycemic carbs? Diet and exercise should be directed at increasing natural HGH. HGH is inhibited by insulin and is contraindicated to excess insulin.

Ratios of HGH to insulin determine ratios of lean body mass to body fat.

High HGH ratios to insulin result in lean muscularity, while low ratios of HGH to insulin result in excess body fat. Foods high in the glycemic index raise blood sugar, which triggers insulin to be released by the pancreas, which in turn causes calories for carbs to be stored as body fat.

So **high glycemic carbs inhibit HGH and exacerbate the storage of fat.**

High glycemic carbs can also cause reactive hypoglycemia evidenced by weakness and fatigue. The glycemic index rates foods according to their ability to raise blood sugar levels. **Low glycemic carbs do not interrupt HGH release or add fat calories.**

Why haven't we heard about the glycemic index before?

The American Diabetic Association and doctors working in the field of diabetes have been using the glycemic index for almost 20-years. The index has been updated in 1986, 1990 and 1991.

How does the glycemic index relate to my muscle to fat ratio?

When you ingest carbohydrates, the pancreas secretes insulin. Conversely, when you ingest protein, the pancreas releases glucagon. It is insulin's job to remove sugar form the blood by pushing it into cells. Excess sugar overwhelms the pancreas and the sugar is simply "swept under the rug" by putting into fat cells. In attempting to promote muscle size and strength gains, too many high glycemic carbs and sugars are generally consumed. When too much insulin is released due to eating too many high glycemic carbs, the body becomes overly efficient in storing calories. When this process occurs over and over, the body does not easily relinquish its fat stores. A good HGH precursor formulation should contain: L-Arginine, 100% free-form, 6 grams per serving, 30 servings to a bottle, 667 mgs of choline, branched chain aminos, fructose, boron, pantothenic acid (B-5), calcium pantothenate, chromium polynicotinate. Note: cannot contain L-Lysine or any other protein.

Foods Low in the Glycemic Index

☆   Apples

☆   Applesauce

☆   Asparagus

☆   Baked Beans

☆   Barbecue Ribs

☆   Beef

☆   Black-Eyed Peas

Blueberries

Broccoli

Buttermilk

Cabbage

Cantaloupe

Cauliflower

Celery

Cherries

Chicken

Chickpeas

Cucumber

Dried Peas

Egg Roll

Fried Chicken

Fried Fish

Garlic

Grapefruit

Grapes

Green Beans

Green Chilies

Green Peppers

Honey Dew Melon

Ice Cream

- Kidney Beans
- Leeks
- Lemon
- Lentils
- Lettuce
- Lima Beans
- Lime
- Milk
- Mushrooms
- Nuts
- Oatmeal
- Oranges
- Peaches
- Peanuts
- Pears
- Pepper Steak
- Plums
- Pork Rinds
- Radishes
- Raspberries
- Red Bell Peppers
- Sauerkraut
- Scallions

- Seeds
- Snow Peas
- Soy Beans
- Spinach
- Sponge Cake
- Squash
- Steamed Fish
- Strawberries
- Sweet Potato
- Tangerine
- Tomato
- Yogurt (Frozen)
- Zucchini

Foods Neutral in the Glycemic Index

- Bacon
- Butter
- Cheese
- Coffee
- Egg Whites
- Ground Beef
- Hot Dogs

- Jell-O
- Lamb
- Olive Oil
- Parmesan
- Peanut Butter
- Pork Chops
- Sausage
- Seafood (Not Fried)
- Steak
- Tuna
- Turkey
- Venison
- Vinegar
- Whole Eggs

Foods Moderate in the Glycemic Index

- Artichokes
- Avocado
- Beets
- Chocolate Milk
- Colas
- Cookies
- Mayonnaise

- Orange Juice
- Pasta
- Pastries
- Pineapple
- Pita Bread
- Pizza
- Raisins
- Spaghetti
- Sugar
- Watermelon
- Wheat Tortillas

Foods High in the Glycemic Index

- Banana
- Brown Rice
- Candy
- Carrots
- Cereal
- Corn
- Corn Chips
- Glucose
- Honey
- Oat Bran

☆ Pancakes And Syrup

☆ Parsnips

☆ Potato

☆ Potato Chips

☆ Puffed Rice

☆ Rice Cakes

☆ Rolled Oats

☆ Wheat Bread

☆ White Bread

☆ White Rice

Chapter 8 - Candida Albicans

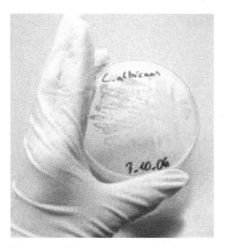

The world is a very tough place. Each and every one of us lives in a sea of bacteria. Infectious agents, known as microbes, swim daily throughout our bodies. Microbes can reside in our throat, mouth, gums, nose, gastrointestinal tract, etc. These microorganisms (i.e., bacteria, viruses, and fungi) are as much a part of every human being as foods and chemicals that we ingest daily. Figuratively speaking, they are constantly trying to "eat us alive". Sometimes they succeed! Even if we die of causes other than infection, they eventually eat our physical remains. Only healthy cells, tissues and organs within our bodies can effectively defend against infectious microorganisms and these make up what is called our immune system.

Microbes, whether they are bacteria, viruses or fungi, do not usually cause illness until an individual's host resistance declines. "Host resistance" is a technical term used by physicians to describe the complicated mechanisms by which our bodies fight off infections. One of the most important defense mechanisms is the destruction of invading microorganisms by blood leukocytes (white blood cells). These special cells actually ingest microbes and render them harmless. But before leukocytes can be manufactured in the body, there must be an optimum supply of amino acids, vitamins A, C, B1, B2, B6, B12 biotin, niacinamide, pantothenic acid and others as well as a complete balance of all minerals and trace elements. If even a single amino acid is deficient or missing, leukocyte production is diminished or may even cease. When this occurs, host resistance within the body is weakened and a greater susceptibility to infection of all kinds ensues.

Another host resistance defense mechanism is the antibody system. When our bodies are receiving optimal nutritional support, specialized protein substances known as antibodies are produced. These substances are constructed from chains of amino acids (proteins). Antibodies also attack invading microorganisms and render them susceptible to destruction by the leukocytes. An individual infectious microbe always provokes antibodies that are specifically targeted against that particular type of microbe and no other. Once the body has synthesized specific antibodies, the lymph cells can reproduce them any time they are needed, provided there are optimum levels of amino acids, vitamins, minerals, trace elements and enzymes from which they can be constructed. Accordingly, if your antibodies for measles, for example, have been synthesized, you will more than likely remain free of measles upon re-exposure to the measles virus. In such a case, your host resistance (i.e., a healthy immune system or adequate production of antibodies, leukocytes and phagocytes), maintained via optimum nutritional support, is functioning properly.

It is essential to understand, therefore, that in the real world, infectious illness occurs not because some "germ" arbitrarily decides to attack our bodies. Rather, illness occurs because our nutritionally deficient, debilitated bodies permit these microbes to set up residence. In short, an opportunist microbe is an infectious agent that produces disease only when the circumstances are favorable.

Nutrient deficits can severely impair the integrity of a healthy immune system. Other factors, however, are also critically involved in resistance to infection. The ingestion of large amounts of sugar, for example, paralyzes the phagocytic capacity of our white blood cells. Likewise, when you fail to obtain your needed quota of sleep, resistance to infectious invasion decreases. Similarly, a personal loss, chronic constipation or diarrhea, irritative chemical exposures to respiratory epithelium, anxiety, too much physical stress, chronic food-chemical allergies and other factors can all influence your resistance to infections. Yet underlying all of these possible causes of poor health are specific nutrient deficiencies, which must be individually tested and diagnosed, and then treated according to empirical laboratory findings.

Traditional medical treatment for bacterial infections flare-up is the administration of antibiotics. Usually little or no advice is given to the patient concerning nutritional support for weakened resistance. And although traditional treatment generally involves drugs that allay symptomatic disorders, the use of drugs does not cure the underlying nutritional-metabolic deficiencies, which are usually the fundamental cause of the illness in the first place. To be sure, this is not to argue against the use of antibiotics. At times, they are very helpful and necessary. However, if the nutritional root causes of infectious disease are not treated, illness after illness may continue to occur, and often become worse, as time goes on. To make matters more disquieting, typical antibiotic medical treatment aimed at the symptomatic relief of infectious flare-up does in fact sometimes produce serious side effects in the form of fungal disorders. The microorganism Candida Albicans is one prevalent example of an infectious overgrowth resulting from the repetitive use, or misuse, of antibiotics.

In its current incarnation, Candida seems to strike women more often than men. Because of the warm, moist condition of the vagina, that is the area most commonly affected. As is the case with all other forms of infection, a compromised host resistance is the primary cause of Candida Albicans. The problem occurs when there is an abnormal fungus, yeast, growth that is normally controlled by friendly bacteria in the intestines. When factors such as antibiotics, steroids (like cortisone), birth control pills and refined sugar are used in excess, friendly bacteria and/or specific nutrients in the blood are destroyed. Host resistance is then lowered and the yeast fungi begin to invade and colonize the body's cells, tissues and finally the organs. A strong, healthy immune systems will, of course, contain Candida's growth. When colonized, these yeast fungi release toxic chemicals into the blood and cause such varying symptoms as yeast vaginitis, rectal itching, chronic diarrhea or constipation, menstrual cramps and irregularities, bladder infections, lethargy, headaches, acne, severe depression, anxiety, nervousness, mental confusion and others. Toxic chemicals produced by the Candida fungi attack the immune system, permitting the fungi to continue their tissue invasion and to cause more serious symptomatic disorders.

Diagnosis

In order to confirm the presence of candidiasis, one must have a high index of suspicion of the condition. Recognition of the risk factors that predispose one to Candida overgrowth is helpful. These are:

☆ Pregnancy or multiple pregnancies.

☆ History of taking birth control pills.

☆ Diabetes mellitus.

☆ History of taking cortisone (corticosteroids).

☆ History of taking antibiotics, especially those of the tetracycline type.

☆ Chemotherapy, irradiation, prolonged illness, debilitation, malnutrition, indwelling catheters, hyperalimentation.

☆ A diet high in sweets, fruits, and juices.

☆ The presence of multiple food allergies and chemical sensitivities.

Candidiasis is the medical term used to describe the yeast fungus overgrowth. It is by no means a new medical problem. In fact, it has been around for centuries. However, candidiasis has become a chronic modern medical dilemma that seems to be increasing rapidly. The reasons for this are the declining vitality of many persons because of several generations of sub optimal diets and the associated factors of drug and chemical exposures.

Treatment

Treatment of candidiasis can involve four major steps: First, the yeast fungi must be killed using a drug called Nystatin. Second, all immuno-suppressive drugs and antibiotics must be used only when necessary. Third, the diet can be altered to deprive the yeast of food upon which it flourishes. Fourth, and most important of all, the body's weakened nutritionally based immune system must be strengthened and thus restored to its proper function. Other forms of treatment are available for those who either cannot tolerate Nystatin or wish not to take the drug. Ketoconazole is a broad-spectrum antifungal drug. Natural treatments include:

 Douche twice a day with a mixture of one-pint water to which is added 4 aqueous chlorophyll capsules and 1 tablespoon of vinegar.

 At bedtime, insert 2-Zymex wafers in the vagina and wear a pad to keep them in place. Zymex wafers contain a strain of yeast known as lactic acid yeast that inhibits Candida.

 Lactobacillus acidophilus organisms can also be inserted in the vagina to counter Candida. Care must be taken that only potent live cultures of Lactobacilli are used,

 Intervaginal use of herbs can also effectively combat vaginal Candida infection. One such herbal powder consists of a mixture of squaw vine, chickweed, slippery elm, comfrey, yellow dock, golden seal, mullein and

marshmallow. These treatments must, of course, be undertaken only with the permission and supervision of a physician.

☆ Garlic also kills Candida. Garlic can be taken fresh or in the odorless form orally. Olive oil and the B vitamin biotin also suppress Candida.

☆ Low carbohydrate (20%)/high protein (50%)/high fat (30%) diet.

☆ Prohibition of all foods containing yeast such as cheeses, bread, sour cream, buttermilk, beer, wine, cider, mushrooms, soy sauce, tofu, vinegar, dried fruits, melons, and frozen or canned juices.

☆ Inclusion of flaxseed oil (four 1000 mg gel caps) taken in the morning and the evening.

☆ A mineral supplement chelated to amino acids only.

Chapter 9 - Healthy Facts for Healthy Living

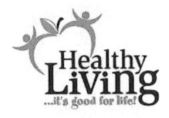

- ☆ Using apple cider vinegar for athlete's foot and jock itch. Simply spray it on or rub it on and wait until dry. When dry, vinegar has the same "ph" level as your skin so it is odorless. Be careful not to get it on your clothes or you'll smell like a Caesar's salad.

- ☆ Put vinegar in your dishwasher and buy the least expensive dishwasher soap. Vinegar is a great grease cutter and dries spot free.

- ☆ Use lemon juice to make your fingernails whiter. The lemon juice actually bleaches them white.

- ☆ Crawling insects hate the smell of bay leaves. Place them in your drawers and cupboards.

- ☆ Basil plants repel insects and flies. Place them in your house and enclosed patio.

- ☆ Rats and mice hate steel wool. Use it to stuff into holes and crevasses that they can enter through.

- ☆ Use tin foil around your plants to keep most animals away from them.

- ☆ Mice hate the smell of peppermint. Place oil of peppermint on a rag and put it in your cupboards.

- ☆ Ants hate the smell of whole cloves, cucumber peelings and Ivory Liquid Soap.

To unclog a drain, use vinegar and baking soda and then stand back for some quick action.

Baking soda added to dishwater cuts grease on dishes and is very inexpensive.

By placing an ice cube overnight on carpet that has been matted down by furniture, it will cause it to be back up by morning.

Flat club soda is excellent for plants.

Warm vinegar will remove most decals. Allow it to soak in for a few minutes.

To take the dents out of ping-pong balls, place them in hot water for 15-20 minutes.

For a smoother texture and longer life, nail polish should be stored in the refrigerator.

Pantyhose will last longer if you freeze them before wearing.

Eating a piece of bacon that does not taste salty is an indication that you are eating too much salt.

If you get migraine headaches, avoid aged wine and cheeses.

If you want clear ice cubes, boil the water first.

To make your hair shiny, try adding a teaspoon of vinegar in your final rinse.

Vinegar makes a great rust and mildew remover from chrome.

Use old milk cartons for large ice cubes. The bigger the cube, the slower it melts.

Apple seeds, plum pits and apricot pits are the most dangerous toxic fruit seeds.

There are 110 pesticides used on apples alone.

Pectin, found in most citrus fruits, is effective in lowering cholesterol.

In a recent study, the chemical called solanine was found effective against arthritis pain. Foods containing solanine are green potatoes, tomatoes, red and green peppers, eggplant and paprika.

Parsley is effective in overcoming bad breath.

The sugar content found in most beans cause intestinal gas.

Soybeans and broccoli are the most nutritious vegetables.

To determine if a mushroom is safe or poisonous, sprinkle salt on the gills. If it turns yellow, it is poisonous; if it turns black it is safe.

If you chew gum while peeling onions, you will not cry.

If you hate the taste of vitamins, store them in the refrigerator but never freeze them. Freezing them crystallizes some of the nutrients rendering them inert.

PMS robs the body of vitamin C.

Breast cancer rates are highest in areas with the least amount of sunshine. Lack of vitamin D could be the problem.

Beta Carotene is only available from plants. Vitamin A comes from animal sources.

Never take vitamin C and aspirin together. Studies indicate that when combined, heavy doses produce excessive stomach irritation, which may lead to ulcers.

The lowest quality meat and poultry is used in canned goods, frozen foods and TV dinners.

Depleted soils are the result of farming only using fertilizers that only replace minerals crucial to crop growth such as phosphorous, potassium and nitrates.

 Smokers require 40% more vitamin C.

 Eating foods high in fat makes you full longer. Approximately 10 grams of fat is cleared from the stomach per hour. Two eggs, bread and butter, coffee and milk equals 50 grams of fat. Assimilation takes 5-6 hours.

 One pound of charcoal barbecued meat contains as much carcinogens as the smoke of 15 cigarettes.

 The average person consumes 129 gallons of fluid per year. For optimum health, 64 ounces (1-gallon) of pure water should be consumed each day for total water consumption alone of 365 gallons per year.

 The colder the water we drink with our meals, the slower the digestive process.

 It takes 5-gallons of water to produce 1-gallon of milk, 100,000-gallons of water to produce one car and 280-gallons of water to print 1-copy of the Sunday newspaper.

 47% of our nation's water supply goes for food production.

 2/3 of all US households are drinking water that violates EPA standards.

Americans spend over $2-Billion/year on bottled water and almost the same amount on filtration and purification systems.

70% of Americans are concerned about the quality of their drinking water.

In a 24-hour period, 55-tons of caffeine and 985-tons of alcohol are consumed in the US.

Approximately $50 Million worth of Twinkies were sold in the US in 1990.

- Americans drink 4,848 cups of coffee every second of every day.
- The average American consumes 1800 pounds of food per year.
- Food manufacturers spend $4 Billion for advertising each year.
- Over a billion pounds of chemical additives are consumed every year.
- White bread may have as many as 16 chemical additives just to keep it fresh!
- When grocery shopping, the highest profit items are placed at eye level.
- Check the bottom of lettuce. If the ring is brown, do not buy it. It should be white.
- Foods on the lowest shelves are usually the least expensive.
- The most commonly purchased items are usually found in the center of an aisle.
- In one year, the average American consumes 100 lbs. of refined sugar, 55 lbs. of fats and oils, 300 cans of soft drinks, 200 sticks of gum, 18 lbs. of candy, 5 lbs. of potato chips, 7 lbs. of popcorn, 63 dozen doughnuts, 50 lbs. of cakes and cookies, 20 gallons of ice cream, 209 lbs. of vegetables, and 149 lbs. of fruit.
- Americans eat approximately 6 pounds of chemical additives per year. The liver is the major organ that has the job of breaking down and disposing of all this material. If certain nutrients necessary to break them down are not available, problems will occur.
- Pasta products are considered a low-fat food and are easily digested due to their low fiber content. Perfect for babies!

Having trouble estimating pasta amounts? Remember this: one cup of uncooked pasta equals two cups of cooked pasta.

 To obtain the right amount of water to cook rice without measuring, place the uncooked rice in the pan and shake it to level it. Add water until it is one inch above the level rice.

 Decaffeinated coffee is the most harmful to you due to the chemical process used to decaffeinate the beans. If you use decaf, buy only the brands that use the "water" process, preferably the "Swiss Process". Also, brewed coffee is good for you if you use the unbleached brown coffee filters instead of the white filters. White filters contain dioxin. Instant coffee is the best and has 50% less caffeine than brewed coffee.

Chapter 10 - Cholesterol (Current research)

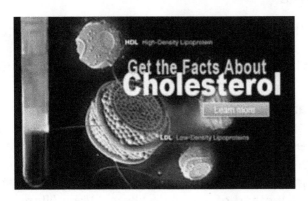

The word itself evokes images of arteries narrowed by atherosclerotic plaque, the gunk that sticks to vessels and impedes the passage of blood the way a kink in a garden hose slows the flow of water.

Or perhaps we think of cholesterol as something our favorite foods—ice cream, two-crust pies, steaks, French fries—are rich in, a culinary spoiler that makes us choose the fish yet again. (Hold the Béarnaise, please.)

But the drumbeat of public health messages about the hazards of too much dietary cholesterol obscures a more complex reality, namely that cholesterol is essential to animal life. I

n fact, much of the cholesterol in us is manufactured by our own bodies, not obtained from our foods. It serves as a precursor to the sex hormones estradiol and testosterone and to vitamin D, which is necessary for the formation of bone.

Cholesterol is also needed to produce the bile acids that digest fats. Cholesterol is only dangerous when the body's regulation of it goes awry, owing to genetic or environmental causes.

The most fascinating aspect of cholesterol is its role in regulating membrane fluidity in animal cells. Far from being simple walls, cell membranes are instead complicated liquid crystals.

About 50 percent of a cell membrane is composed of lipids (oily organic compounds like fats) and most of the rest is made of proteins. The whole lot is characterized by randomness, chaos, and subtlety.

Membranes are not rigid little sheets. They fluctuate, they're dynamical systems, and they are remarkable. The normal fluidity of cell membranes is now thought essential to life functions, and disruptions can have dire consequences.

Just this year scientists reported that cholesterol's regulation of membrane fluidity may be involved in the destruction of brain cells that leads to Alzheimer's disease; that reduced fluidity in the membranes of red blood cells may be related to psoriasis outbreaks; that abnormalities in membrane lipid content may cause resistance to leptin, the hormone that regulates appetite to maintain normal body weight; and that chromium, a carcinogen, causes tumors by reducing membrane fluidity.

Membrane fluidity is probably involved in all cell processes associated with communication of cells with each other and with the outside world. Experimental studies suggest that membrane fluidity and cellular communication are related.

Membranes consisting of the lipid diphenoylphosphatidylcholine and cholesterol undergo a clear phase transition between a gel and a fluid state at a lipid/cholesterol ratio of about eight.

At this and higher concentrations of cholesterol, the lipid is held in a gel-like state by the cholesterol. At lower concentrations of cholesterol, the lipid melts into a fluid state. This observation is significant, because phase change is associated with a significant change in the character of the cell membrane.

The high-cholesterol gel phase is much less fluid than the low-cholesterol phase.

The cholesterol-induced phase change observed in a membrane patch in the computer shows the mechanism for the experimentally observed cholesterol-induced fluidity changes, presumably those associated with the normal processes of cell fusion and perhaps even the pathology of Alzheimer's disease.

Another study looks at the ion channel proteins embedded in cell membranes. These little living batteries convert the chemical potential of ions into electrical currents.

They are essential to intercellular signaling and to transporting material between the inside and the outside of a cell. If scientists can understand these biomolecules on the atomic level—understand exactly how a given protein structure results in an observed current—then it should be possible to engineer ion channels into the workhorses of nanodevices built partly of biological materials.

Eventually the components of highly sophisticated nanodevices might be embedded into such engineered cell membranes.

Such nanodevices would live in the body much like any other cell, taking over functions lost to disease or injury.

Although scientists have already demonstrated the feasibility of building such hybrid nanodevices, much more work is needed before such devices can be successfully installed and function in a living organism.

Chapter 11 – I Have a Special Gift for My Readers

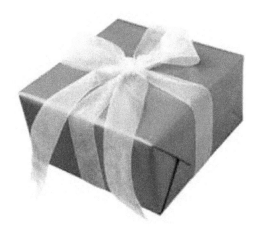

I appreciate my readers for without them I am just another struggling author attempting to make ends meet. My readers and I have in common a passion for the written word as well as the desire to learn and grow from books.

My special offer to you is a massive ebook library that I have compiled over the years. It contains hundreds of fiction and non-fiction ebooks in Adobe Acrobat PDF format as well as the Greek classics and old literary classics too.

In fact, this library is so massive to completely download the entire library will require over 5 GBs open on your desktop. Use the link below and scan all of the ebooks in the library. You can select the ebooks you want individually or download the entire library.

The link below does not expire after a given time period so you are free to return for more books rather than clog your desktop. And feel free to give the link to your friends who enjoy reading too.

I thank you for reading my book and hope if you are pleased

that you will leave me an honest review so that I can improve my work and or write books that appeal to your interests.

Okay, here is the link…

http://tinyurl.com/special-readers-promo

PS: If you wish to reach me personally for any reason you may simply write to mailto:support@epubwealth.com.

I answer all of my emails so rest assured I will respond.

Meet the Author

Dr. Leland Benton is Director of Applied Web Info, a leading Internet Marketing company based in Utah. With over 21,000 resellers in over 22-countries, its operating entity - Neternatives.com - is a leader in Information Technology and online marketing. He is also a behavioral scientist and Chief Forensics Investigator for ForensicsNation.com. Leland resides in Southern Utah.

http://www.amazon.com/author/lelandbenton

Visit some of his websites
http://appliedmindsciences.com/
http://appliedwebinfo.com/
http://bookbuilderplus.com
http://embarrassingproblemsfix.com/
http://www.epubwealth.com/
http://forensicsnation.com/
http://www.freebiesnation.com/
http://neternatives.com/
http://privacynations.com/
http://refernationwordofmouth.com/
http://survivalnations.com/
http://texternation.com/
http://thebentonkitchen.com
http://theolegions.org
http://willilookgoodinthis.com

CPSIA information can be obtained
at www.ICGtesting.com
Printed in the USA
LVHW08s1407021018
592095LV00040B/393/P